The CHRISTMAS HEART

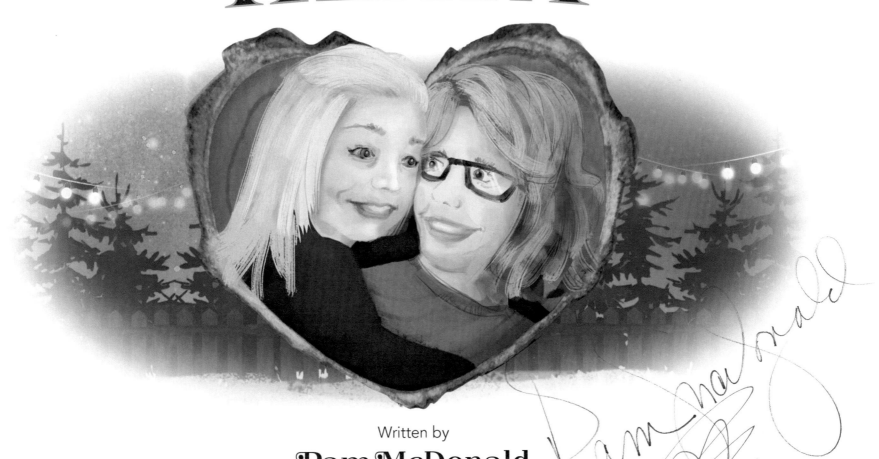

Written by

Pam McDonald

Illustrated by

Kim Hanzo

www.teacup-press.com • www.foxpointepublishing.com/author-pam-mcdonald

Library of Congress Cataloging-in-Publication Data
McDonald, Pam, author.
Eckman, Raven, editor.
Hanzo, Kim, illustrator.
Hanzo, Kim, designer.

The Christmas Heart / Pam McDonald. – First edition.

Summary: A girl shares the story of losing her grandma to Alzheimer's disease, then receiving a sign from her late grandma at Christmas time.

ISBN 978-1-955743-68-6 (hardcover) / 978-1-955743-69-3 (softcover)

[1. Christmas & Advent – Fiction. 2. Death, Grief, Bereavement – Fiction. 3. Disease – Fiction. 4. Grandparents – Fiction.]

Library of Congress Control Number: 2 0 2 3 9 3 1 2 9 0

Printed and bound in the United States of America by Lakeside Press Inc.

First printing May 2023

To my grandchildren:

Lily, Kate, Dalton, Will, Greta, Frederick,
Donavan, Peyton, Vivian, Drake and Chloe

...being your Grammy inspired me to tell another
Grandma's story.

— ◆ —

To my husband, Mike, who always told me
I should write a book.

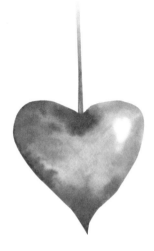

Christmas.

It's my favorite time of year.

We have so many fun Christmas traditions, like baking cookies or getting our trees together as a family.

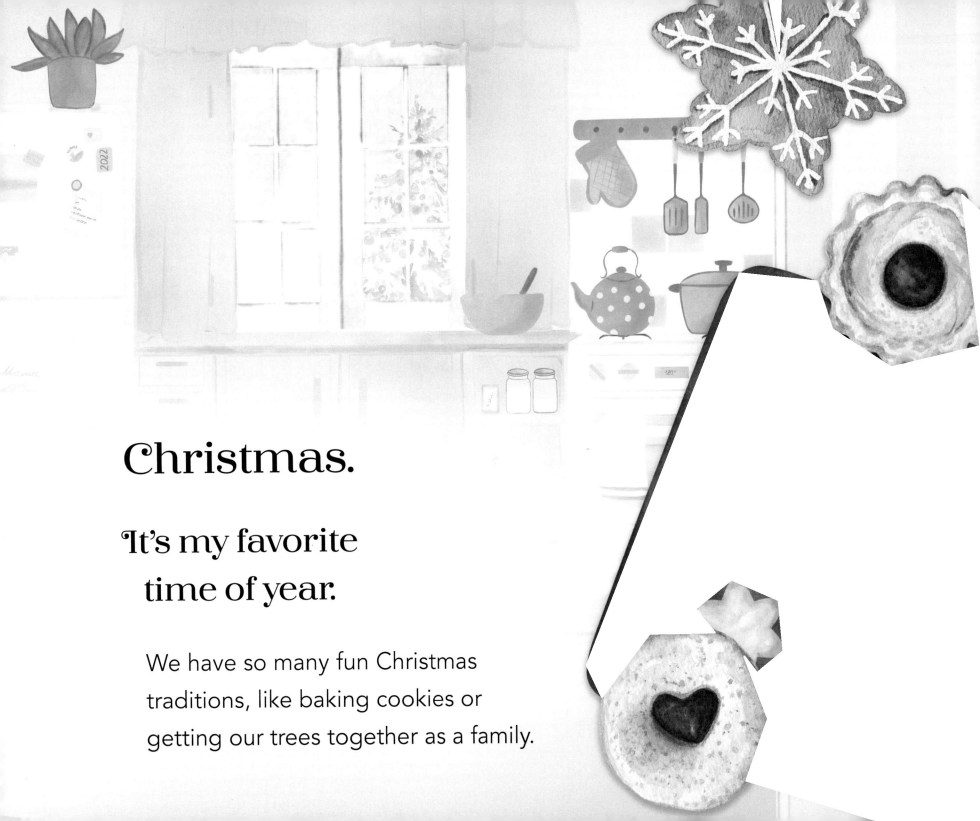

By the way, I'm Madi and Christmas is just around the corner.

It's the Saturday after Thanksgiving and my whole family—aunts, uncles, cousins, and grandparents—are picking out our trees at Goldenman Christmas Tree Family Farm.

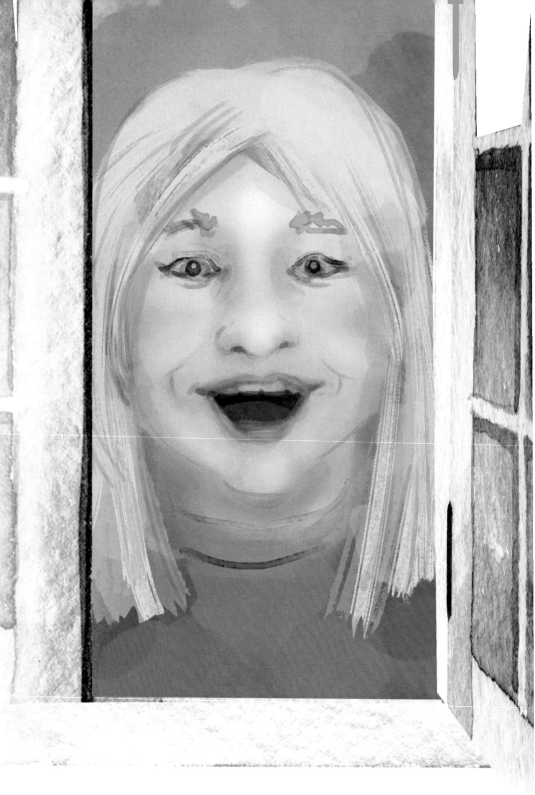

Everyone is looking
for their perfect tree.

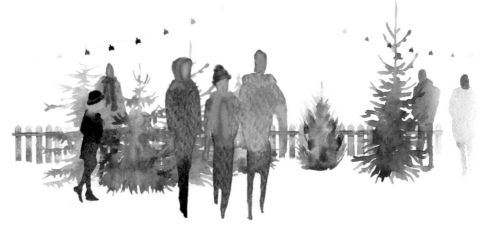

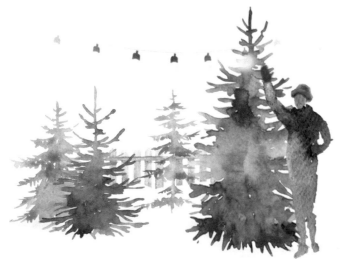

My dad always finds ours first.
He just wants the tree to be big.

Grandpa Mark always
finds his tree last.
He needs the tree to
"speak to him."

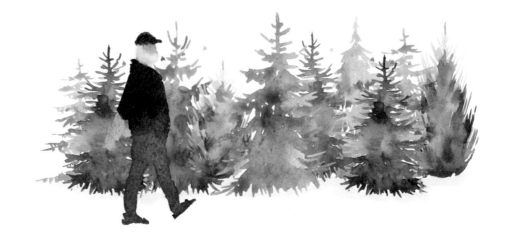

While each year brings a new tree-finding adventure, last year's adventure was one I'll never forget.

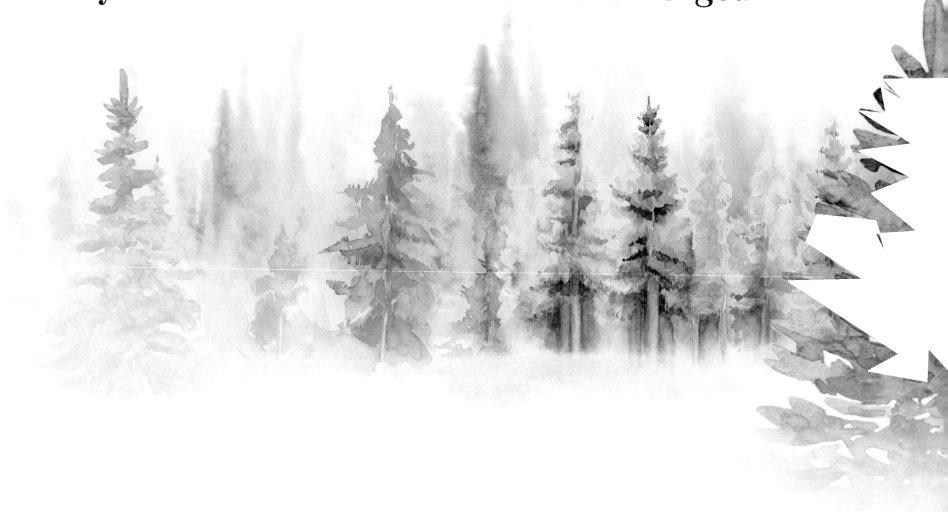

But first, this story started long before last year.

I grew up in Albertville, Minnesota with two younger sisters and two younger brothers. Since taking care of our large family took a lot of time, my Grandma Patti started coming over on Thursdays to help my mom with housework and us kids.

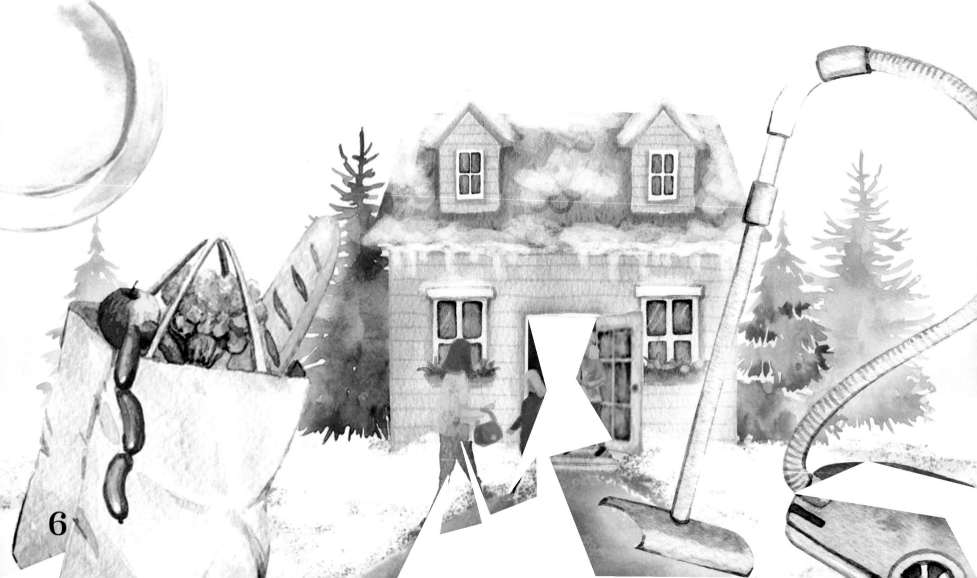

Sometimes Grandma Patti would bring old wooden puzzles and tell us the stories of how my mom and her siblings used to play with them while we put them together.

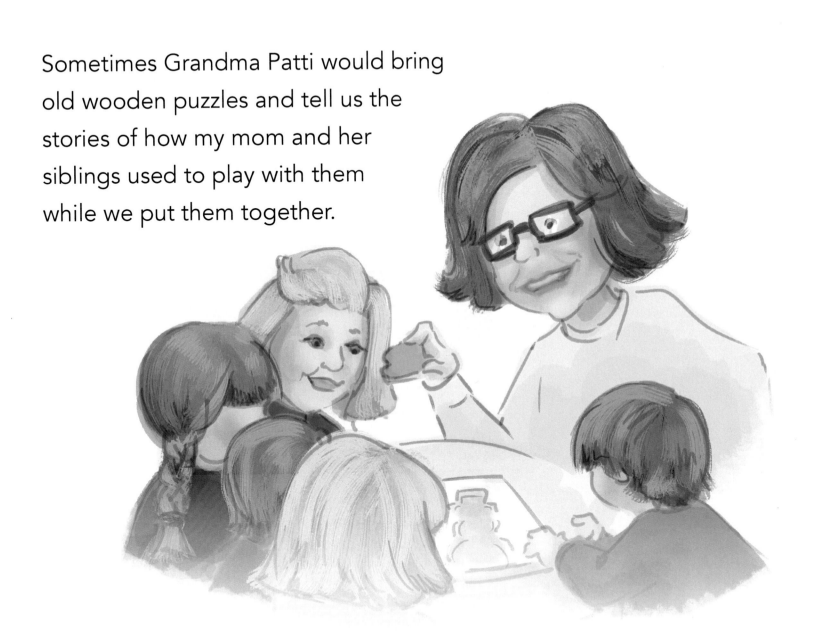

They had an old, musty smell that I loved.

Sometimes we did a craft, like making beaded necklaces. Grandma Patti always added a red heart bead at the end of her necklaces.

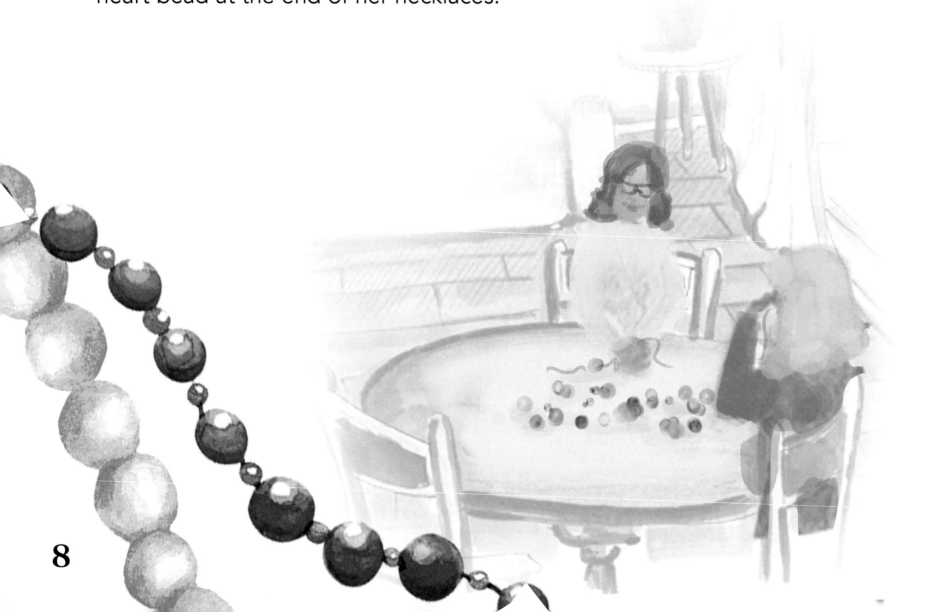

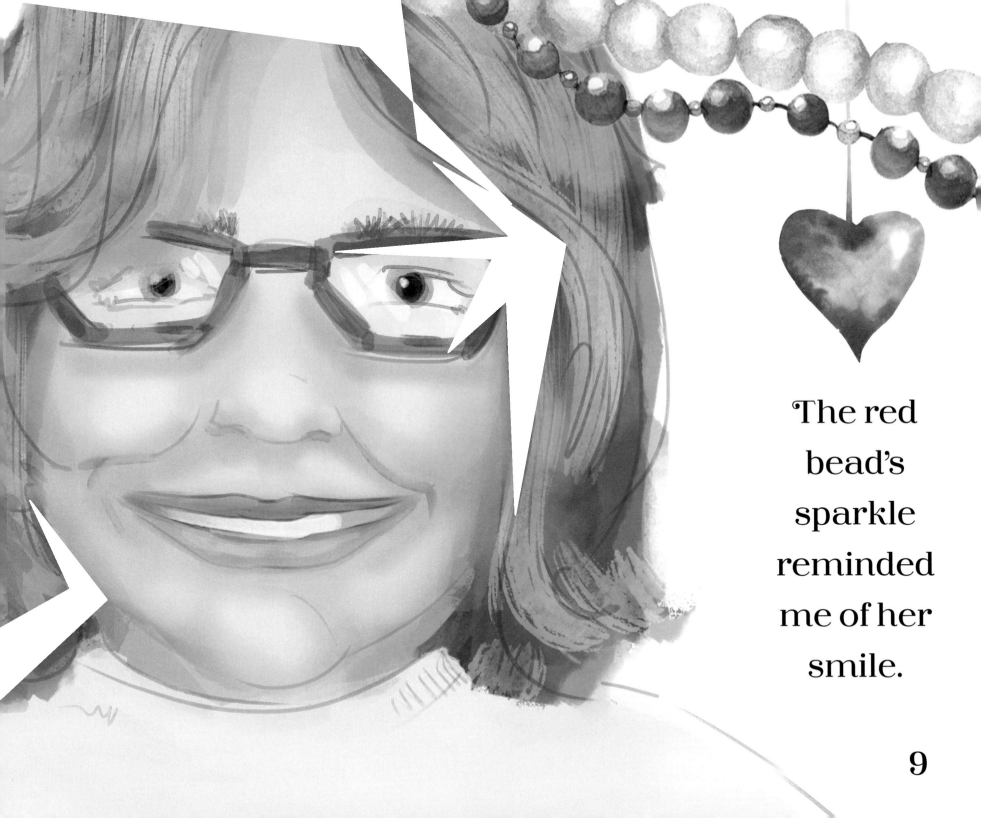

The red bead's sparkle reminded me of her smile.

9

For lunch, Grandma Patti would usually make peanut butter and jelly sandwiches.

She always made a heart when she swirled the strawberry jam on the bread.

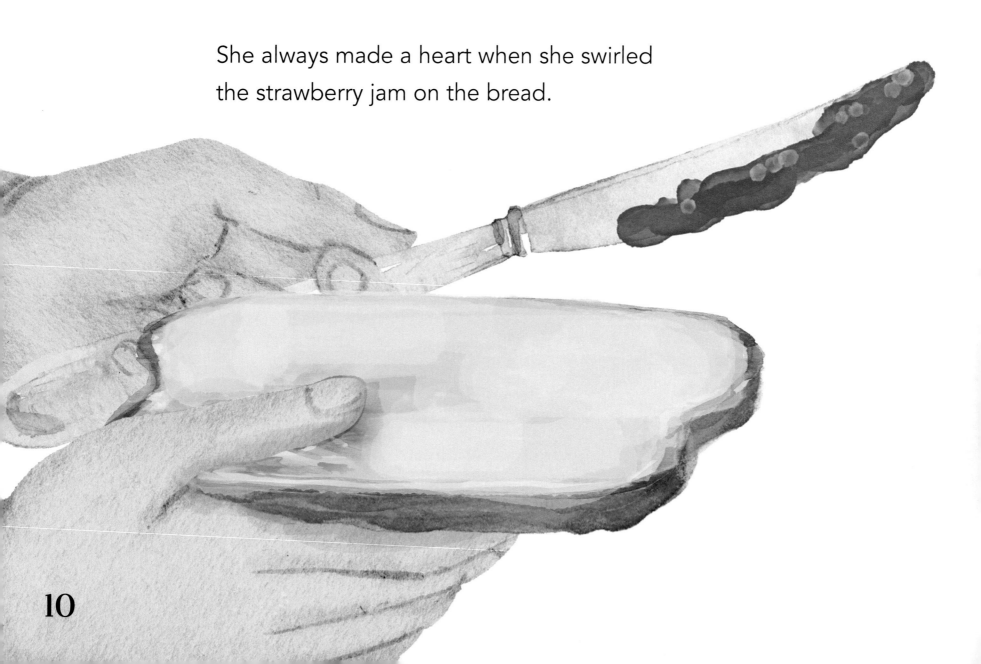

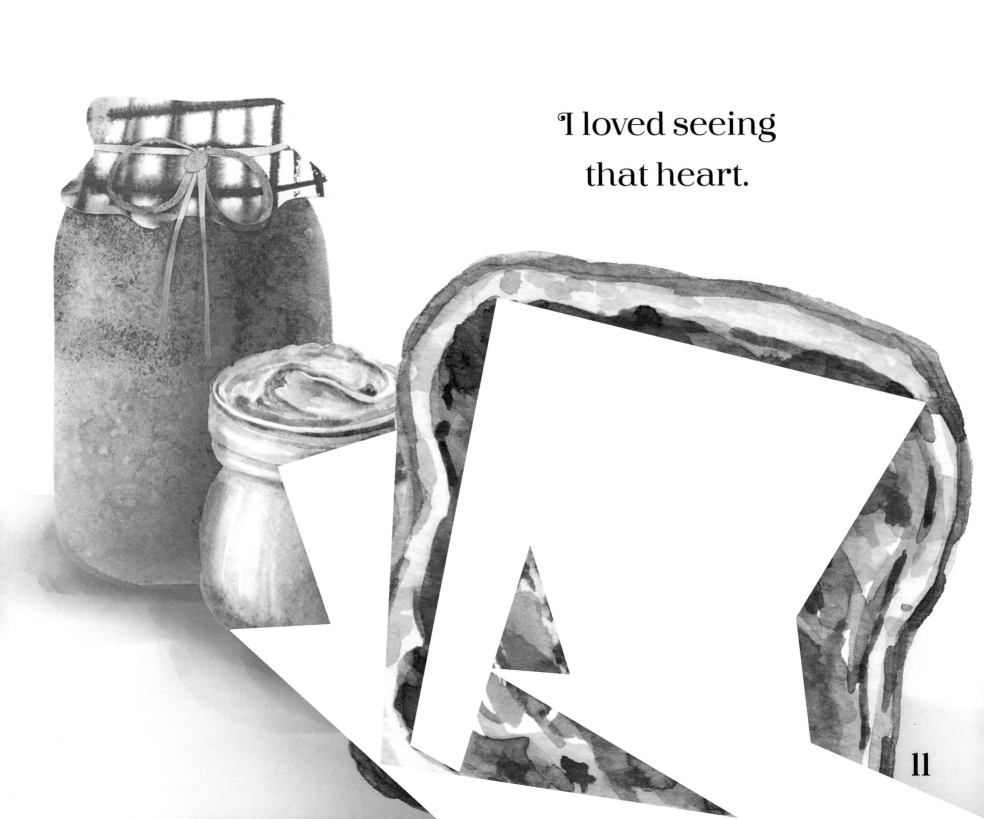

I loved seeing
that heart.

11

Even as I got older and started school, Grandma Patti still came on Thursdays. She would get me on the bus in the morning.

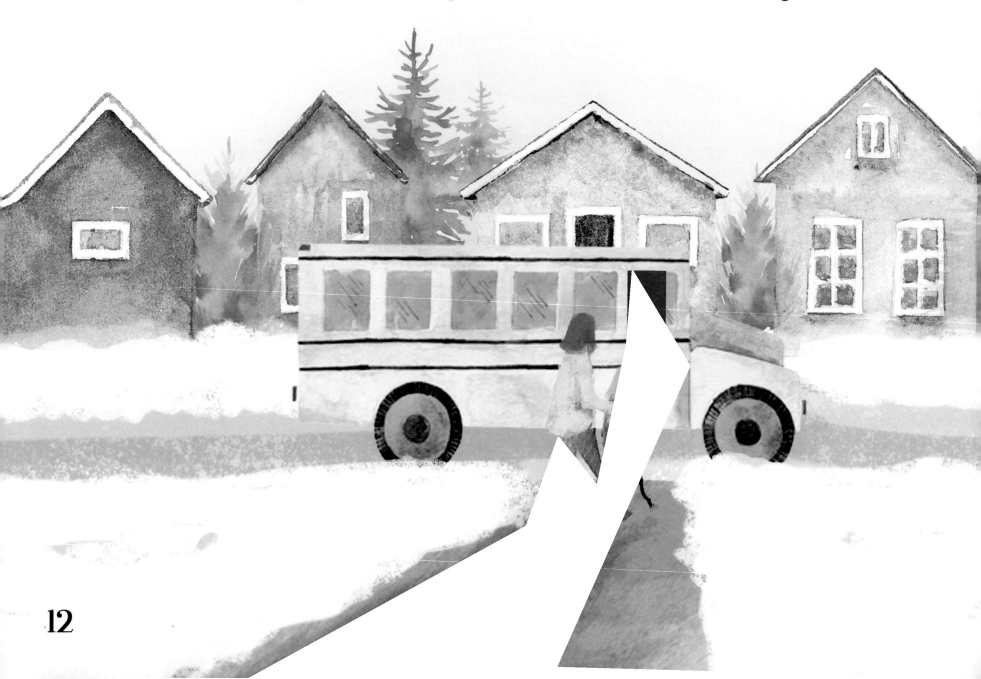

12

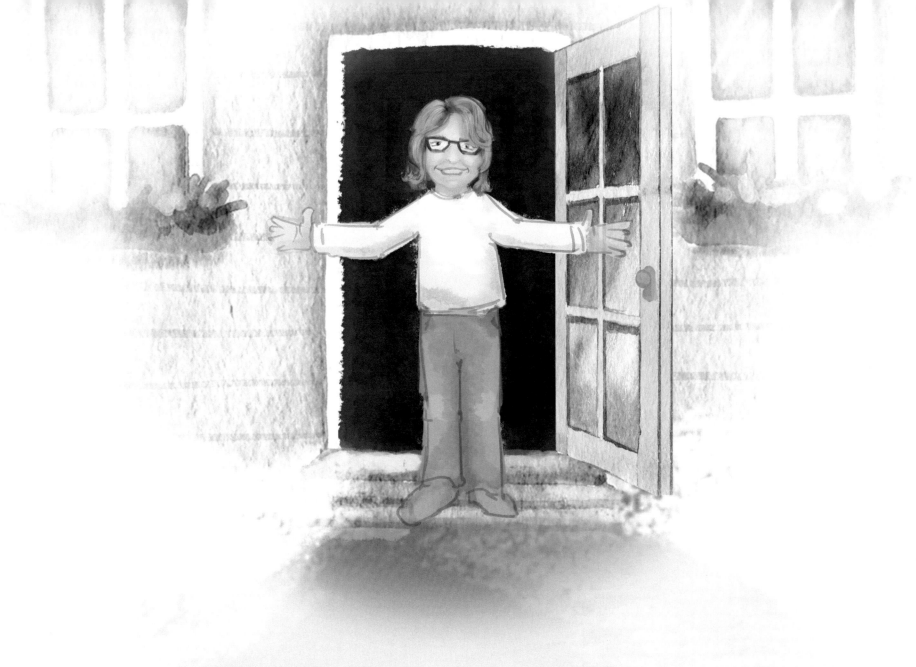

In the afternoon, her sparkly eyes and smile greeted me when I got home.

Life was great, until it began to change.

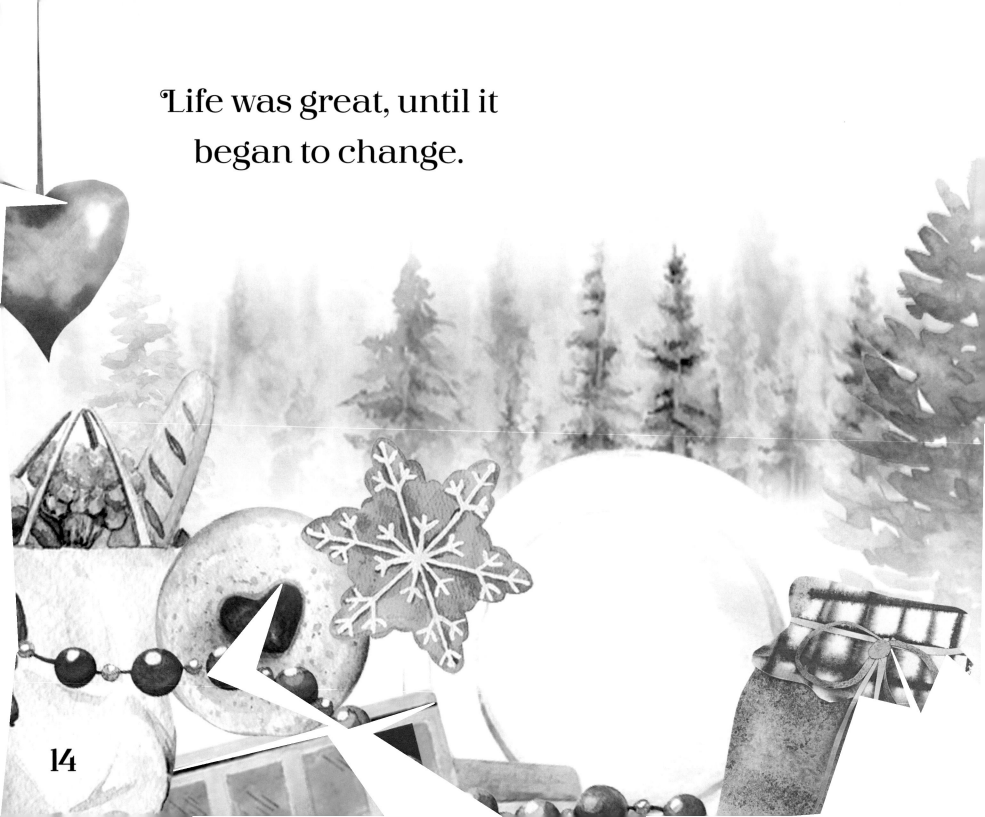

When I was ten, I started noticing that Grandma Patti forgot things. Like forgetting to put jelly on our sandwiches or not remembering where Mom kept the knives.

Other times she couldn't remember where she put her car keys.

The forgetting worried me, but even though she forgot things, she never forgot to smile. It made her forgetfulness seem not so bad.

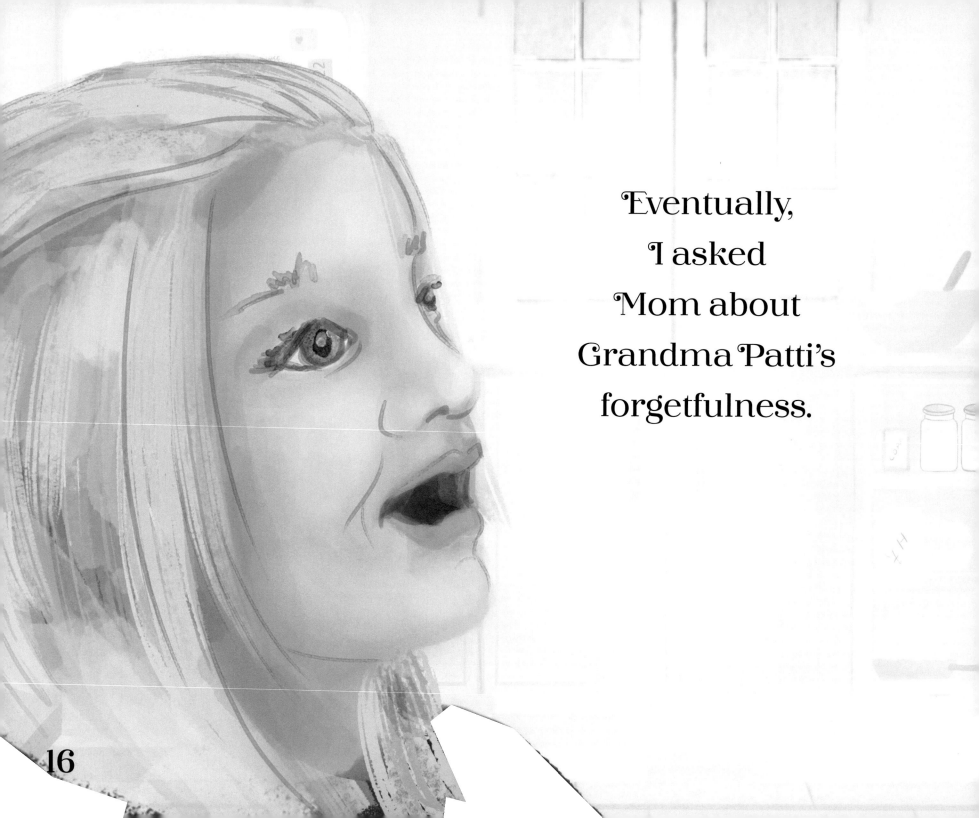

Eventually,
I asked
Mom about
Grandma Patti's
forgetfulness.

16

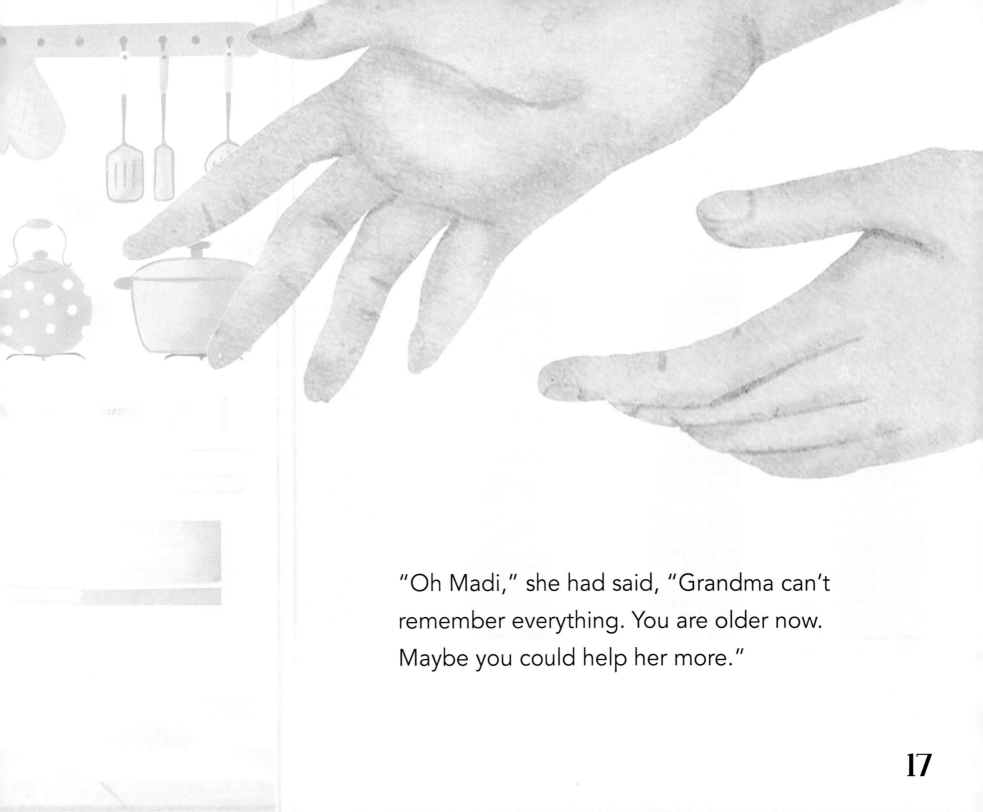

"Oh Madi," she had said, "Grandma can't remember everything. You are older now. Maybe you could help her more."

17

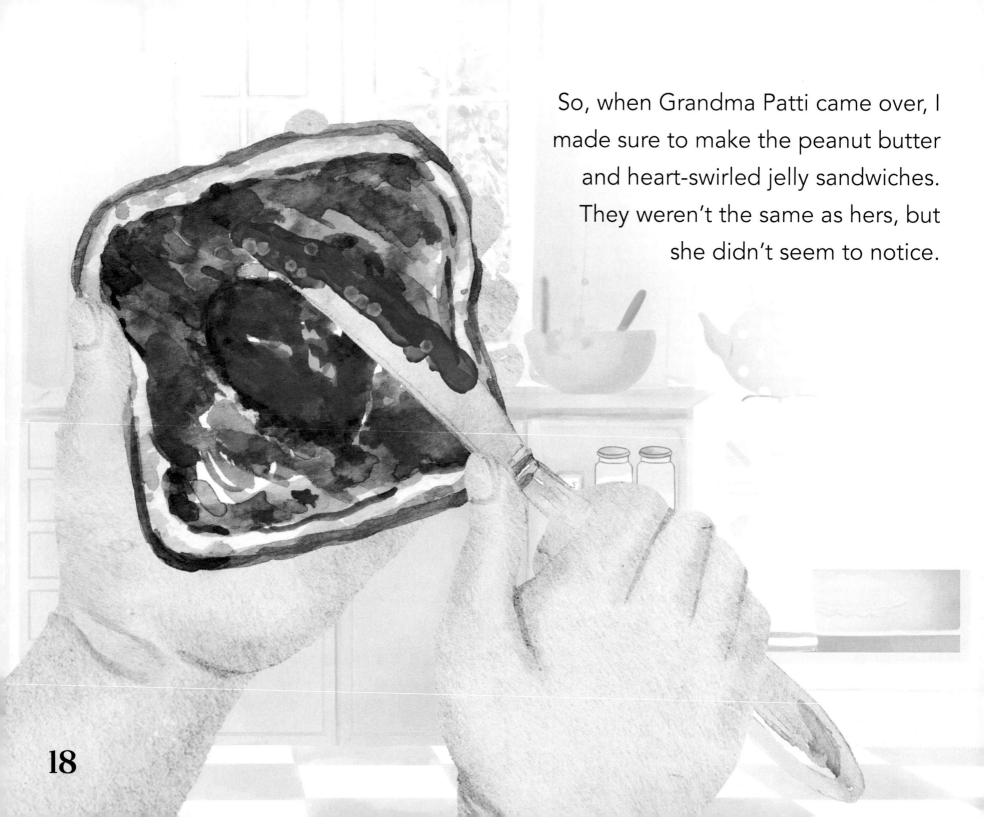

So, when Grandma Patti came over, I made sure to make the peanut butter and heart-swirled jelly sandwiches. They weren't the same as hers, but she didn't seem to notice.

18

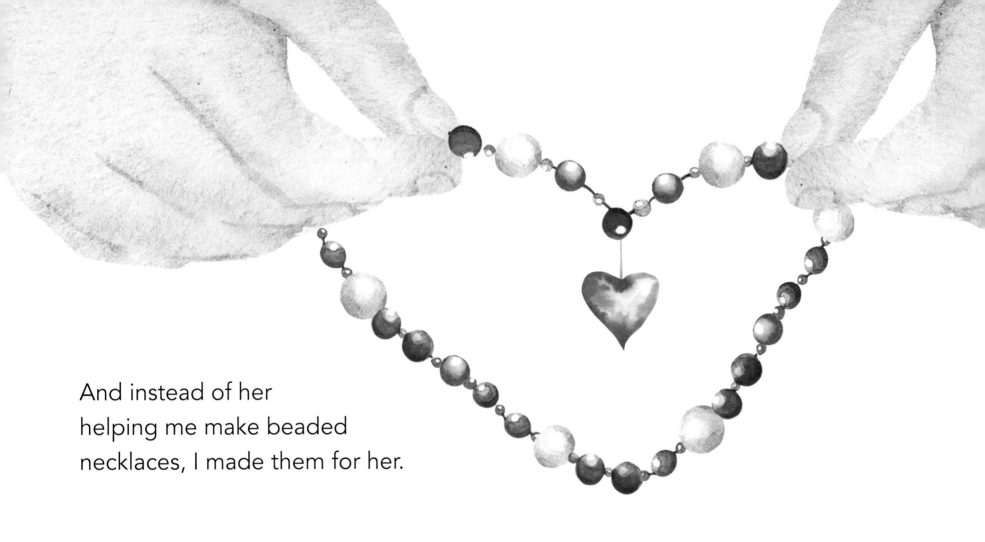

And instead of her helping me make beaded necklaces, I made them for her.

I always remembered to add the red heart bead at the end too.

19

I was so sure my help would make
Grandma remember everything again.

But Grandma Patti still forgot
things…even more things.

Mom and
Grandpa Mark
started to notice.

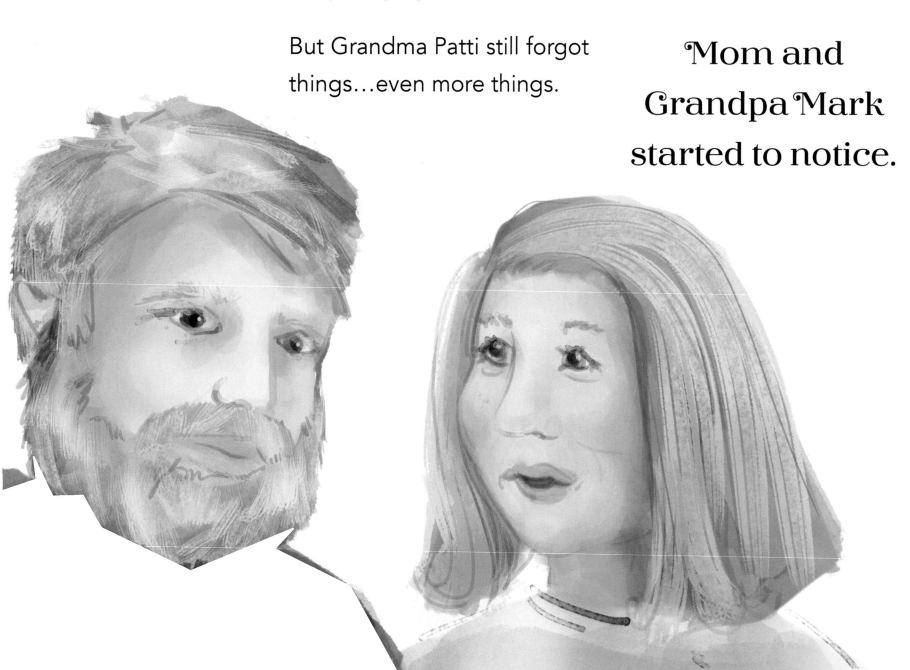

Grandpa Mark took Grandma Patti to the doctor. The doctor said that she had an illness called Young-onset Alzheimer's Disease.

This meant that she would keep forgetting things.

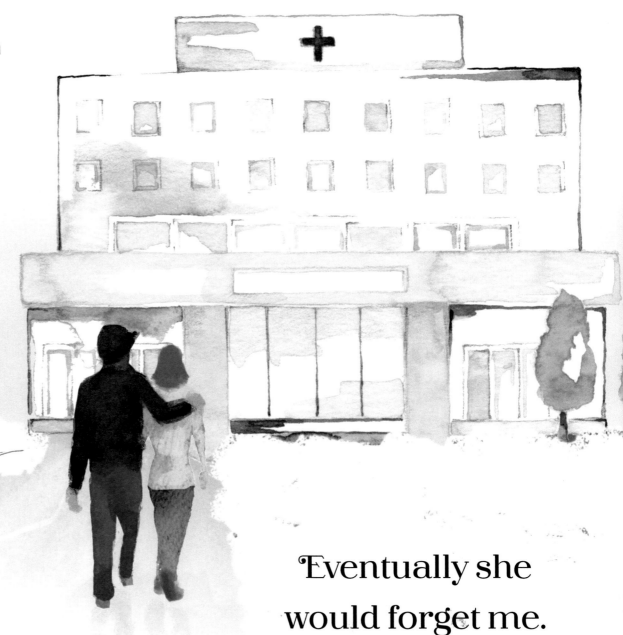

Eventually she would forget me.

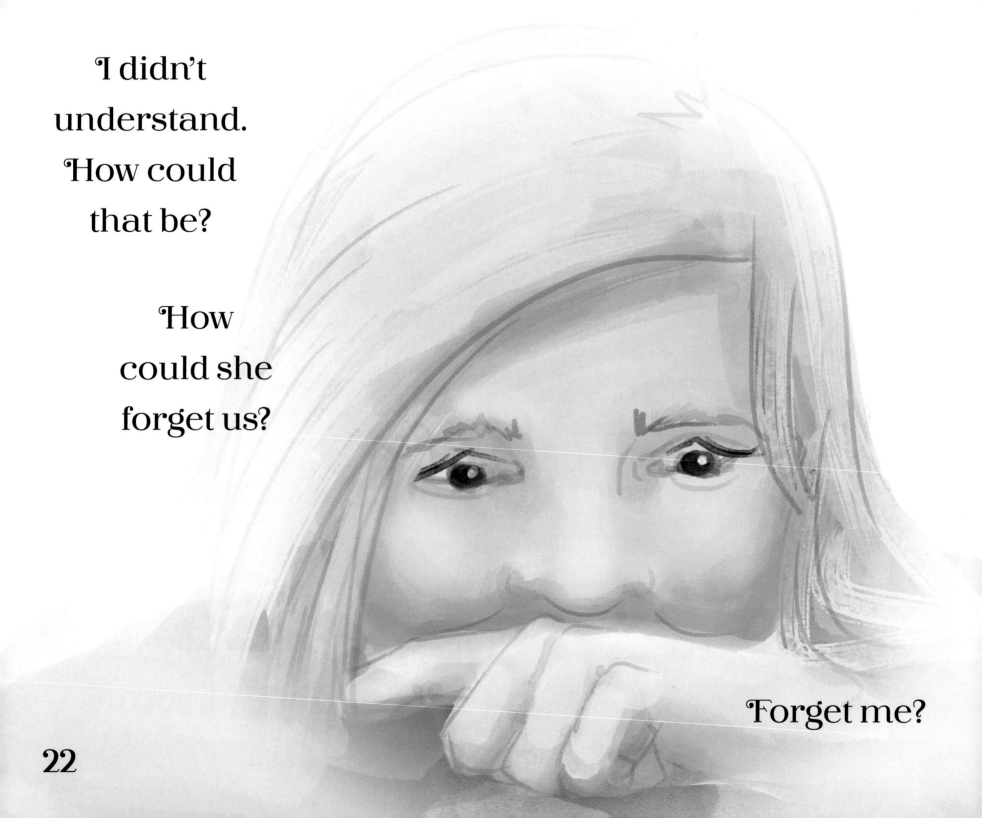

I didn't understand. How could that be?

How could she forget us?

Forget me?

22

Grandma Patti still looked the same.

Her eyes still sparkled.

She still smiled.

But I knew
that she was
changing.

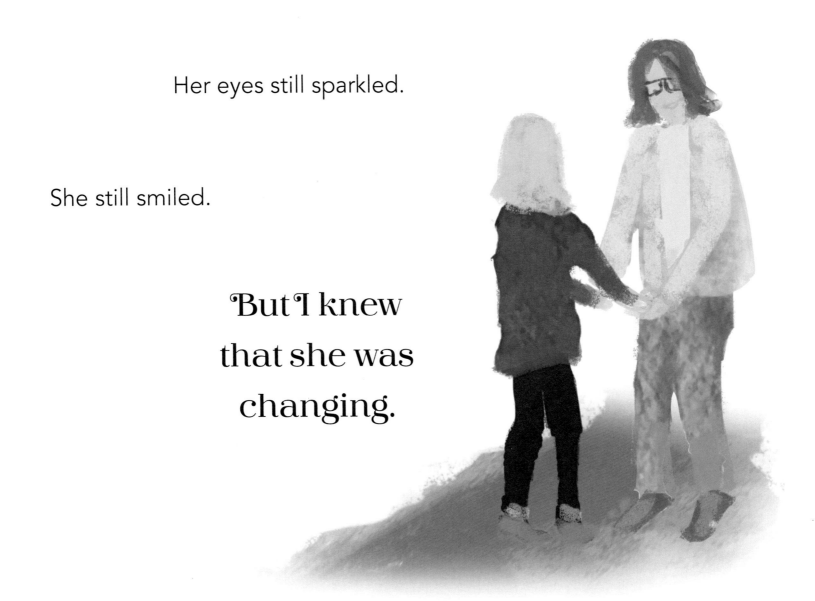

When I was twelve,
Grandma Patti forgot my name.

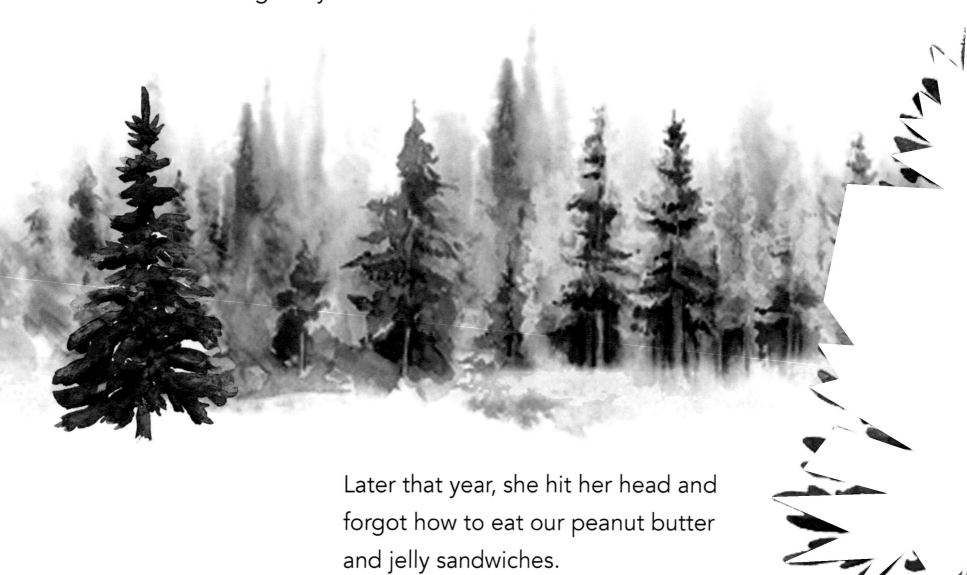

Later that year, she hit her head and
forgot how to eat our peanut butter
and jelly sandwiches.

On a sunny day in late September, Grandma Patti's sparkling eyes and smile left us for good.

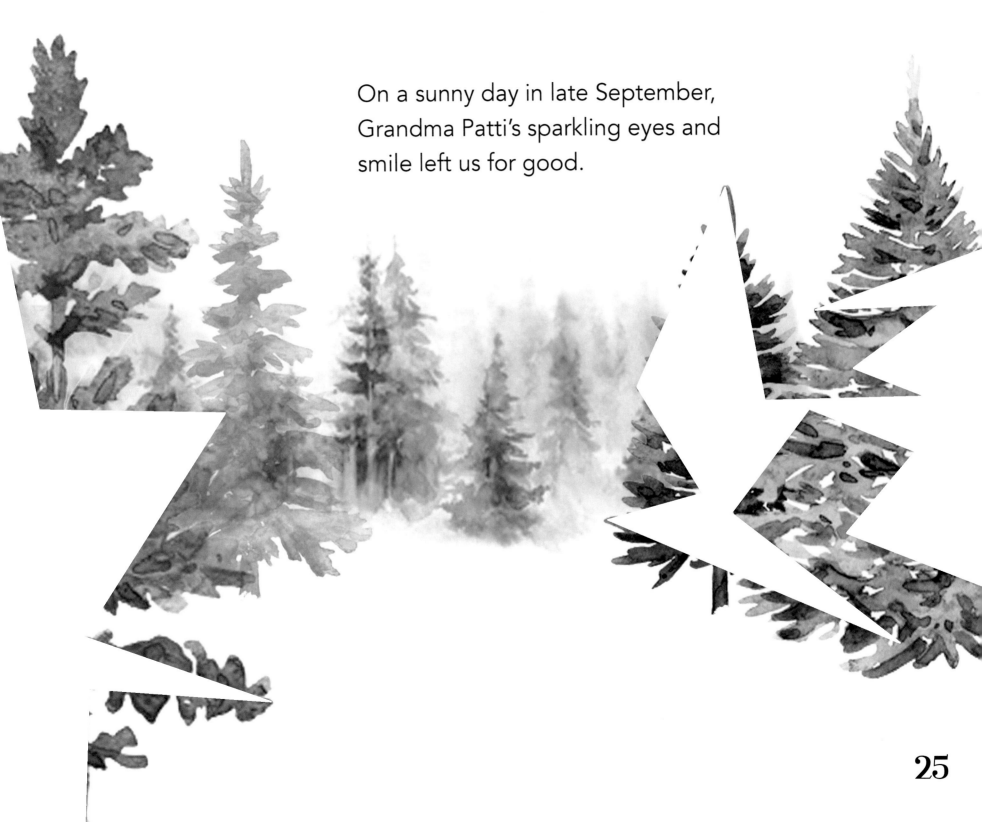

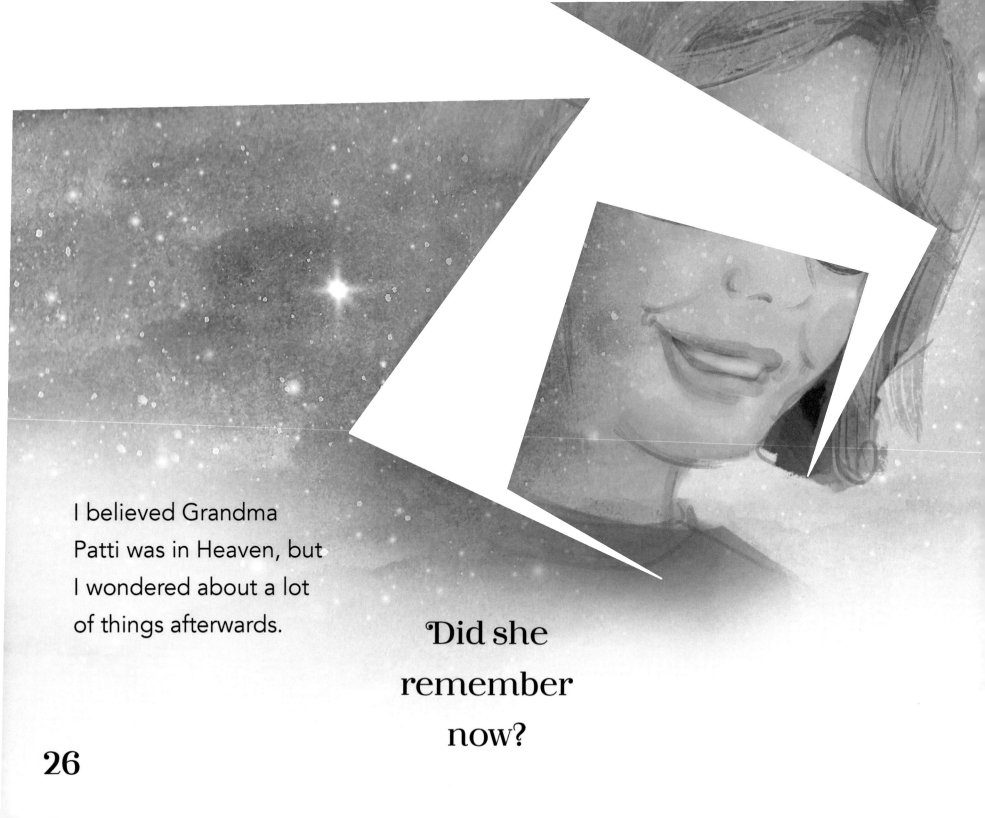

I believed Grandma
Patti was in Heaven, but
I wondered about a lot
of things afterwards.

Did she
remember
now?

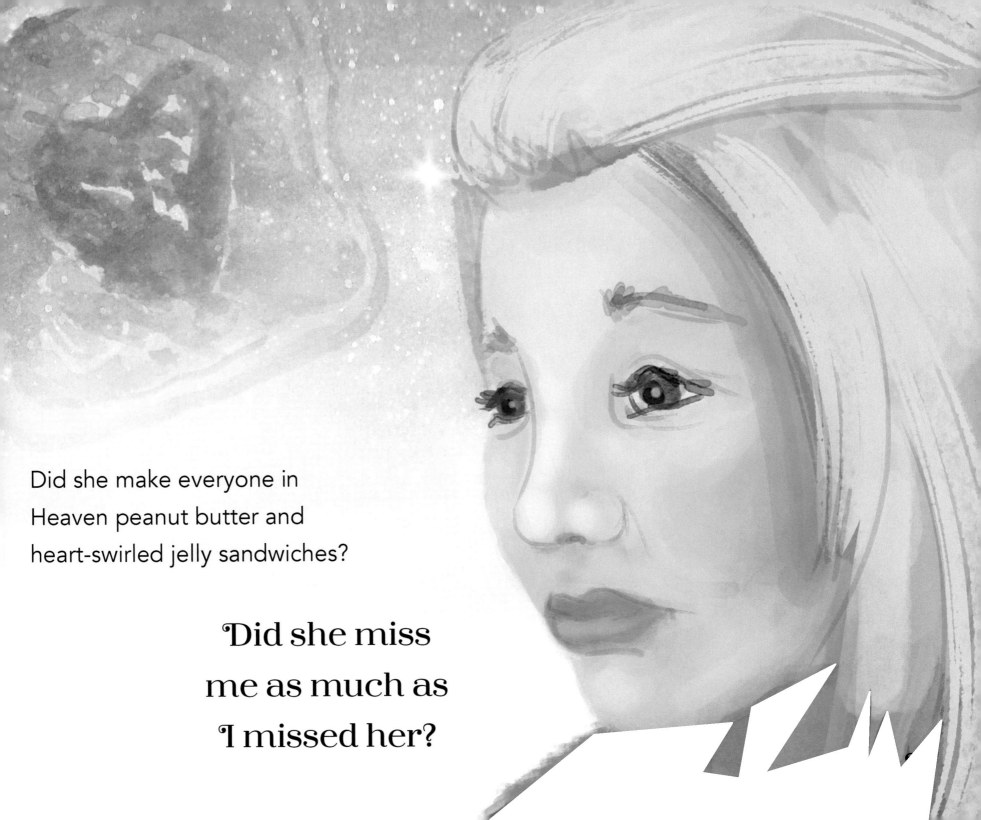

Did she make everyone in Heaven peanut butter and heart-swirled jelly sandwiches?

Did she miss me as much as I missed her?

Halloween came and then Thanksgiving.

Soon it was time to go to
Goldenman's for Christmas trees.

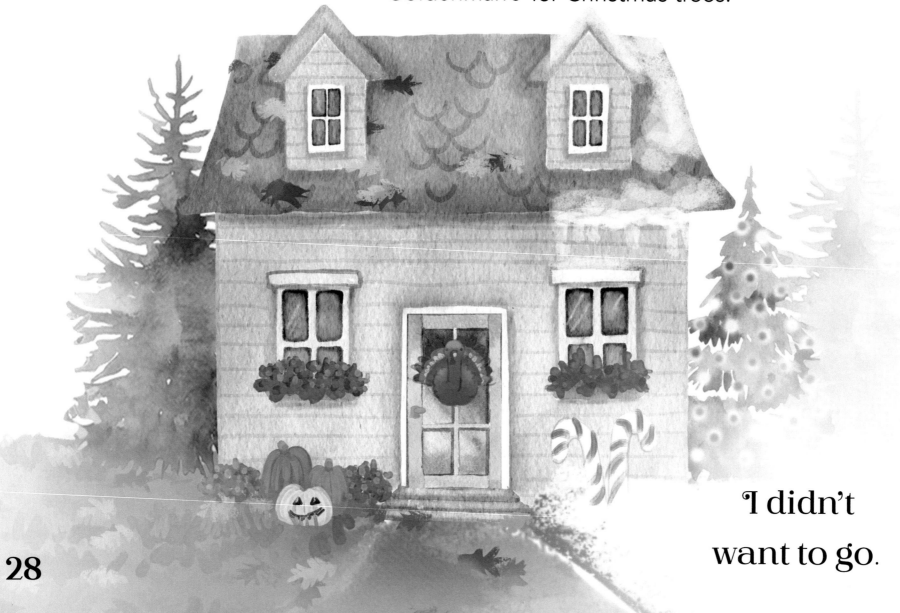

I didn't
want to go.

It would be strange without Grandma Patti,
and I wanted to skip going this year.

But Grandpa Mark said, "This is what our family does."

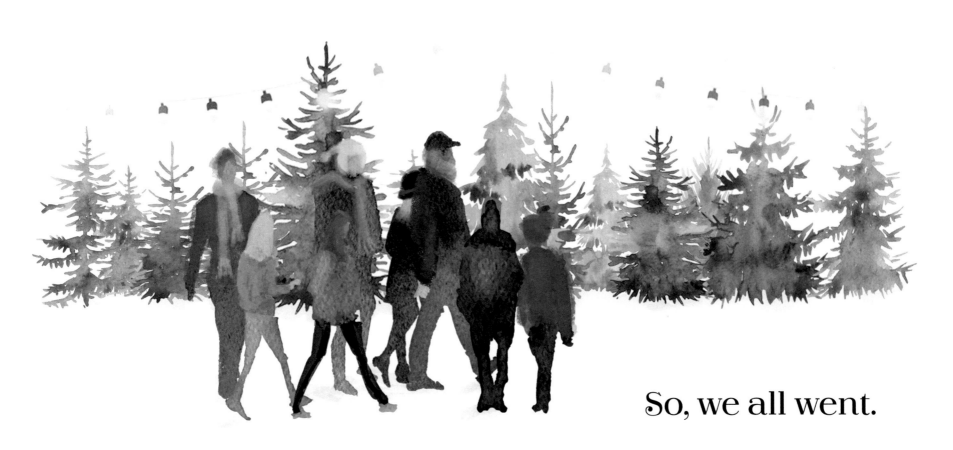

So, we all went.

Once we got to Goldenman's, everything did seem the same.
And, of course, my dad found our tree first.
It was a big one.

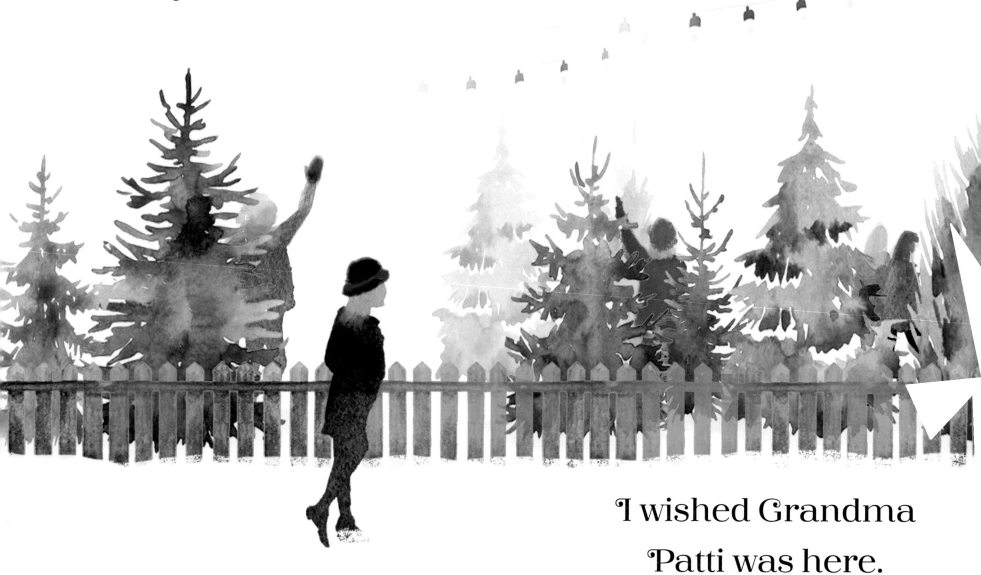

I wished Grandma
Patti was here.

One by one, everyone else found theirs too, except for Grandpa Mark. It seemed like it was taking him longer than usual to find his tree.

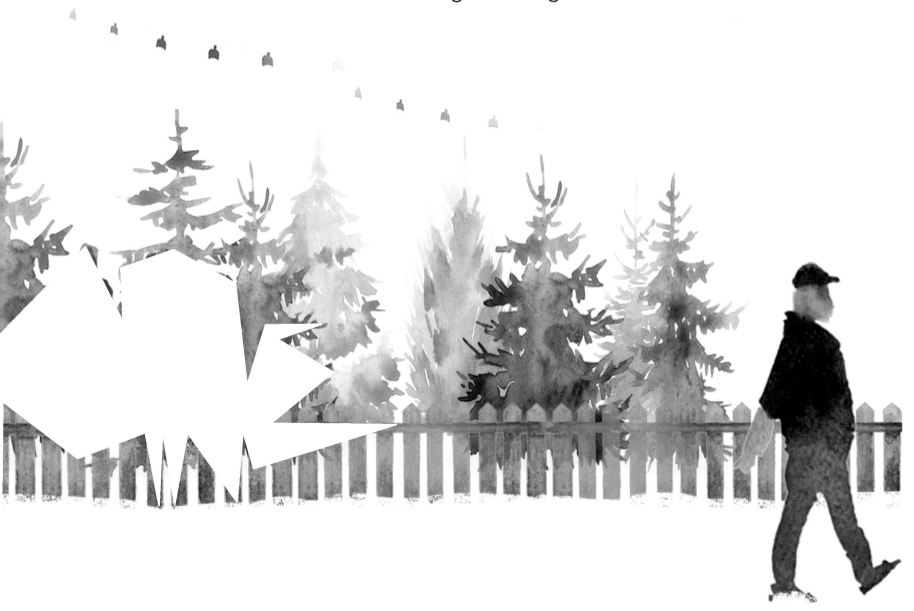

Just when I thought I couldn't stand the cold and the waiting any longer, I heard, "Found it! Over here!"

We were all relieved.

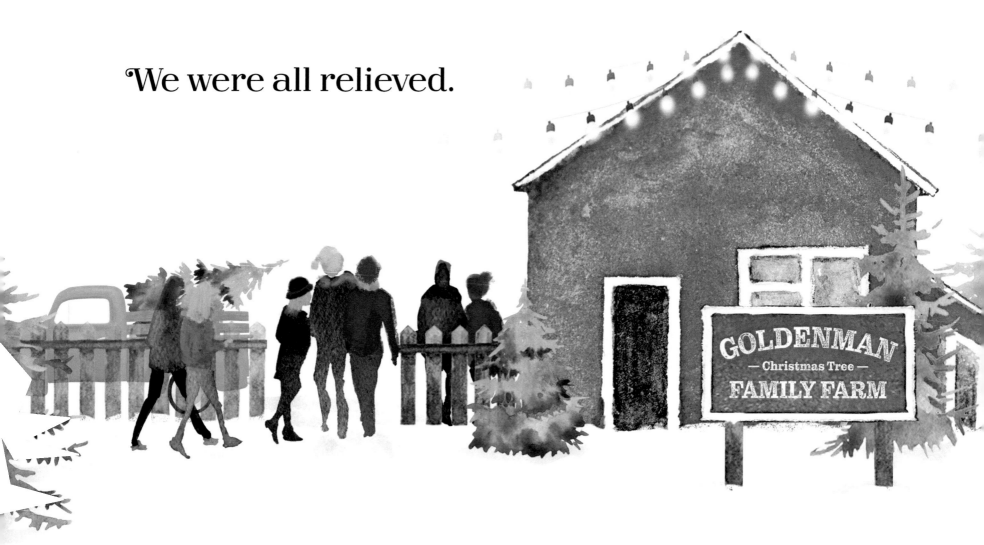

Uncle Patrick ran over with his saw and began to cut down
the tree, while the rest of us waited at the tree farm entrance.

Suddenly Grandpa Mark yelled,
"Everyone! Come quick!"

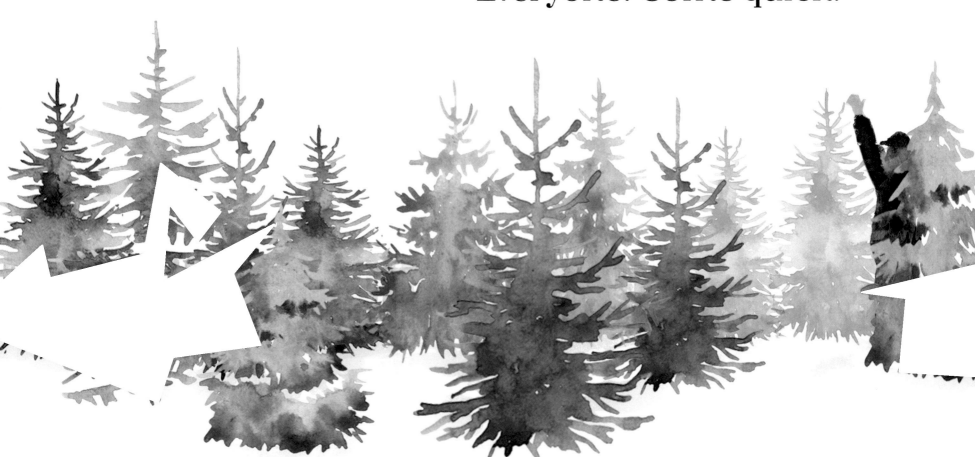

When we got there, I saw it—

The stump from the tree Uncle Patrick had just cut
was in the shape of a heart … a red heart.

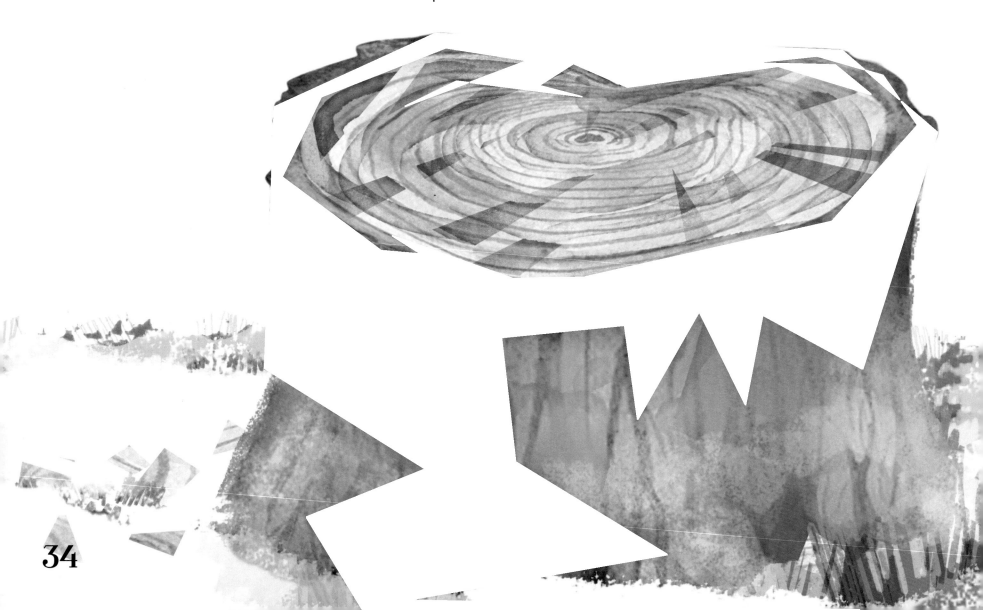

No one said a word.

Grandma Patti was here, smiling up at
all of us from the heart of the tree.

I believed she was letting us
know that she remembered
and was still with us.

Goldenman Christmas Tree Family Farm let us cut out
the tree stump the next day and give it to Grandpa Mark.

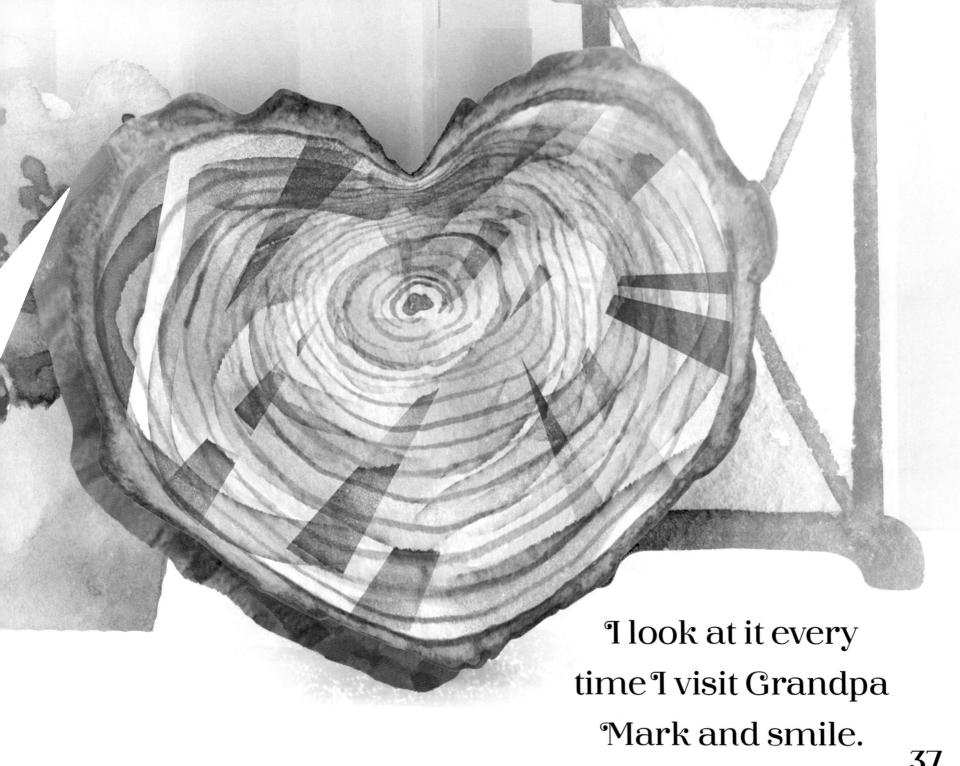

I look at it every time I visit Grandpa Mark and smile.

37

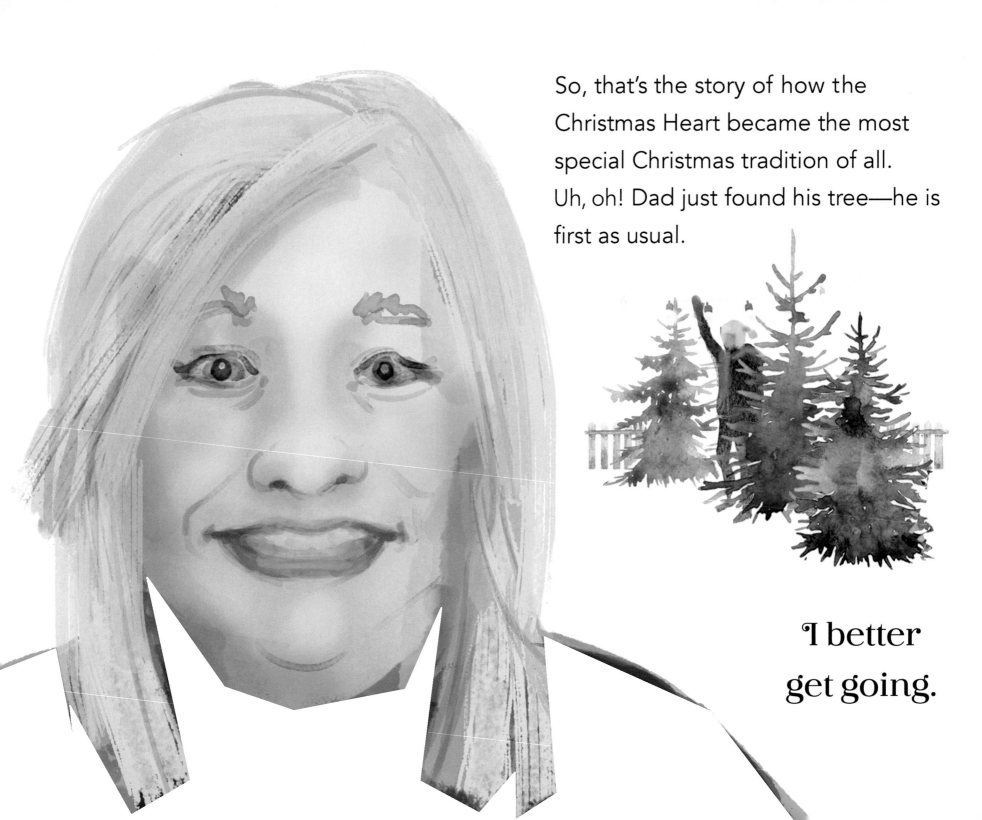

So, that's the story of how the Christmas Heart became the most special Christmas tradition of all. Uh, oh! Dad just found his tree—he is first as usual.

I better get going.

I share a smile with Grandpa Mark
as we walk among the trees.

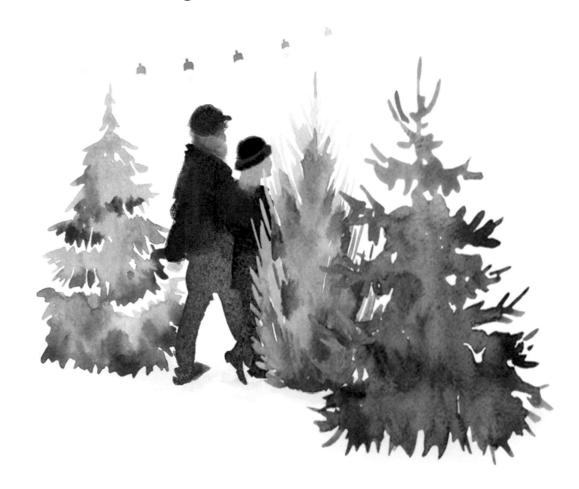

Grandma Patti will always be with us.

About the Author

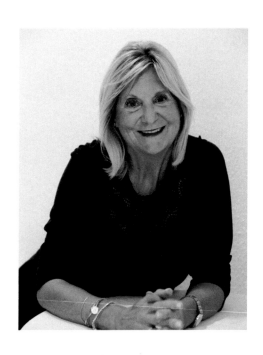

Pam McDonald is a former long time elementary educator. Pam developed her passion for working with children in her hometown of Chicago. She continued that passion as she studied at the University of Illinois and the University of St. Thomas. She has taught in a variety of school districts throughout Illinois and Minnesota. Now retired, Pam spends her days with her husband at Camp McDonald on the shores of Lake Marion in Lakeville, MN. Her best times are spent with all the campers…including her four daughters, their husbands, and her eleven grandchildren.

Acknowledgements

Special thanks to Megan Lawinger for sharing her mother, Patti Schommer's story. Patti's children have started a foundation to support others dealing with Alzheimer's.

For more information, visit: https://humbleandkindalzfoundation.org

Turn the page for a
Christmas Heart ornament!

— ◆ —

Christmas Heart Ornament

With a parent's help, cut out the ornament and paste it to a piece of craft paper or cardboard. Punch the hole out and string a purple ribbon through, then tie the ribbon's ends together.

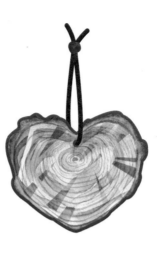

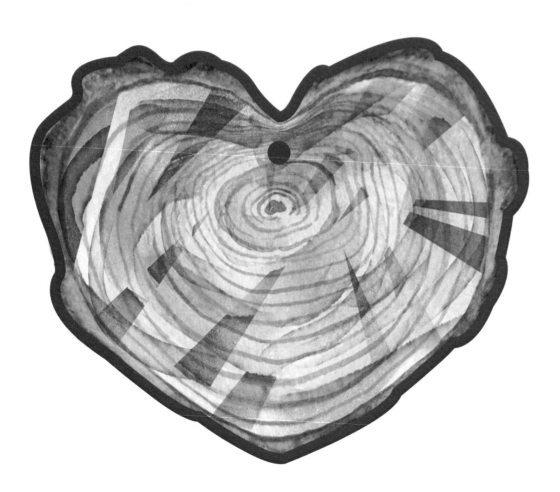